A MESSAGE FOR YOU

MW01070071

WARNING

READ AT YOUR OWN RISK!
EVERYTHING IN THIS BOOK MIGHT BE WRONG...
BUT IT MIGHT JUST FEEL RIGHT.

CANCER ISN'T FUNNY.

THERE'S NO RIGHT OR WRONG WAY TO APPROACH IT,
BUT LAUGHTER HELPS.

YOU CAN'T CONTROL WHAT COMES YOUR WAY,
BUT YOU CAN CONTROL YOUR REACTION.

WE DIDN'T WANT YOU IN OUR CLUB, BUT NOW
THAT YOU ARE, WE'RE HERE TO HELP!

THIS BOOK WAS WRITTEN BY
CANCER ASS-KICKER KIM KOVEL, AND ILLUSTRATED
BY ARTIST-INSTIGATOR MARK SMITH.

KIM & MARK ARE ALSO DESIGNERS AT NIKE,
WHERE THEY LAUGH A LOT AND NEVER COLLUDE.

HEALTH BENEFITS OF LAUGHTER

ACCORDING TO SCIENTIFIC RESEARCH,
LAUGHTER CAN HELP...

LOWER BLOOD PRESSURE
(WE ALREADY HAVE CANCER,
LET'S AVOID HEART ATTACK & STROKE)

BOOST T CELLS
(YOUR IMMUNE SYSTEM WILL APPROVE)

TRIGGER ENDORPHINS
(YOUR BODY'S NATURAL PAINKILLERS
AND YOUR FREE "LEGAL HIGH")

REDUCE STRESS LEVELS
(OHM...)

IMPROVE MENTAL FUNCTIONS
(COMBAT CHEMO BRAIN)

SO LAUGH.
IT'S CONTAGIOUS...
UNLIKE CANCER.

COLORING WHILE LAUGHING MAY LEAD TO
MORE FAMILY TIME, REGULARITY, SPELLS OF CONCENTRATION,
ANNOYING OPTIMISM, QUESTIONABLE COMMENTARY,
CHILDHOOD REGRESSION, AND SOME DAMN
GOOD FUN !

THIS BOOK IS FOR YOU

ANSWER THESE QUESTIONS TO BE SURE
YOU'LL GET THE CORRECT DOSE OF FUNNY.

_____

"WHAT'S YOUR FULL NAME ?"

_____

"WHAT'S YOUR DATE OF BIRTH ?"

_____

"WHAT'S YOUR DIAGNOSIS ?"

EXTRA CREDIT:
HOW MANY TIMES HAVE
YOU BEEN ASKED THESE THREE
QUESTIONS TODAY...

_____

FREE COLORING PAGE!

ALL ABOUT YOU

TAKE A FEW MINUTES TO SHARE A LITTLE ABOUT YOURSELF.

FAVORITE
PLACE _____

FAVORITE
FOOD _____

FAVORITE
COLOR _____

FAVORITE
ANIMAL _____

FAVORITE
BAND _____

FAVORITE
MOVIE _____

FAVORITE
TV SHOW _____

FAVORITE
FRIENDS _____

FAVORITE
MEDS _____

TELL CANCER
SOMETHING... _____

_____

_____

_____

_____

SKETCH YOURSELF
IN A COSTUME

FIND THE LUMP

THE JOYS OF EARLY DETECTION!
THERE'S ONLY ONE LUMP TO FIND...... SEARCH LEFT,
RIGHT, UP, DOWN, FORWARD AND BACKWARD.

```
J A U O T L J Q B Y X I L R H
P V K Q B Z I R S W I B R Y L
A G D M I S E P M U L S L K O
B K H F H Q D J B Q J H T U F
F Z D N G E D C X D K V I F K
J J H T Y G I W I G B U K S Z
L M J L Z J U H H E G J C Y P
O Y A Q C T W P T F I Y V X T
I U I T W D I V R T R Q R N C
G O C G S Z V E U H L A H A T
U E D M P D F N A P X K R R T
B G K G R N P Z X U J H I N J
Z G E F F O N U Z X U I M F N
J Z K I B R G D V D S K E U H
A T I W P N C J X R T L S M B
M Y W X U W X S H P Z S U Z O
G T O R Q R Z E Z K Q V M T I
X W W M A Z J L Y Z I A B G T
J V C U Y M H I Z D C Z C Y M
M W V M Y F X C X N V Y N H X
```

LIST THE INGREDIENTS
IN A CORN DOG

TOP TEN

REASONS TO CATCH CANCER!

RATE THEM 1 – 10

○

PRESCRIPTION WIGS COVERED BY OBAMACARE

○

NO NEED TO SHAVE, OR WAX ...ANYTHING !

○

SKINNY JEANS FIT AGAIN !

○

BALD IS "IN" WITH THE KIDS THESE DAYS

○

"MEDICAL" MARIJUANA

○

MEDICAL GOWNS WITH "EASY ACCESS"

○

"CONVENIENCE" BASED FORGETFULNESS

○

"TASTE" IS SOOOO OVER RATED

○

LATEX GLOVES

○

LEARNING NEW LANGUAGES
(MEDICAL, INSURANCE, SWEARING)

SKETCH YOUR NEXT TATTOO

BRAIN MAZE

CAN YOUR CHEMO BRAIN MAKE IT
THROUGH YOUR FIRST MAZE ?

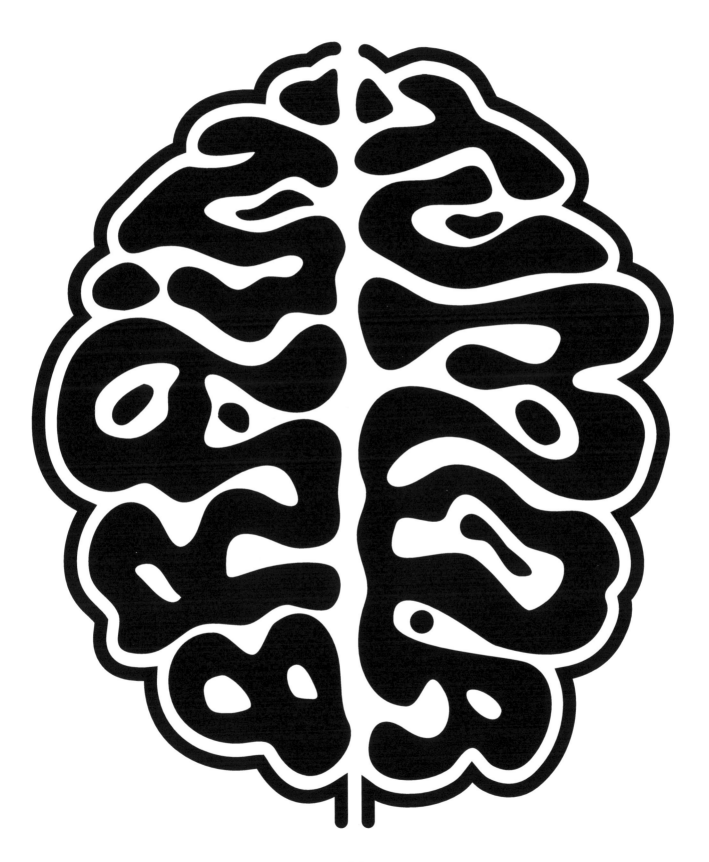

LIST YOUR
FAVORITE DISEASES

TODAY'S CANCER HOROSCOPE

FILL IN THE BLANKS

(TO BE READ VERY MYSTICALLY)

SCHEDULE PLENTY OF _____ OVER THE NEXT _____

NOUN ...... AMOUNT OF TIME
TO REASSESS AND REDEFINE YOUR _____ RATHER THAN

NOUN
LIMITING IT TO THE PRESENT CIRCUMSTANCES.

INSTEAD OF ONLY _____ ON THE _____ WORK YOU

VERB ...... ADJECTIVE
MUST DO TODAY OR _____ OBSESSING ABOUT

ADVERB
_____ , LOOK FOR WAYS TO CULTIVATE YOUR LONG TERM

NOUN
_____ -

PLURAL NOUN

IMAGINE WHERE YOU WANT TO BE IN _____

AMOUNT OF TIME
JUST SO YOU CAN PLAY A TRICK ON _____

FAMILY MEMBER

ULTIMATELY, IT'S MORE SATISFYING TO _____

VERB
YOUR _____ SQUIRM THAN TO

NOUN
YELL AT THE TOP OF YOUR LUNGS... " _____ !"

EXPLETIVE

_____ ARE FOR KIDS...

NOUN
BUT EVERYONE ENJOYS A GOOD _____

ACTIVITY

WRITE A LETTER
TO THE PRESIDENT

DOT TO DOT

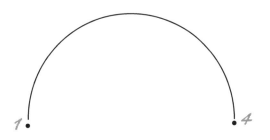

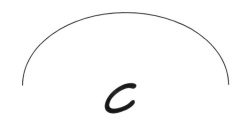

C

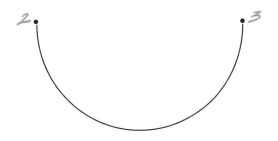

FREE JOURNAL PAGE!

HAPPY HOUR

GRAB YOUR CRAYONS AND CUSTOMIZE
YOUR CHEMO COCKTAIL. CHEERS!

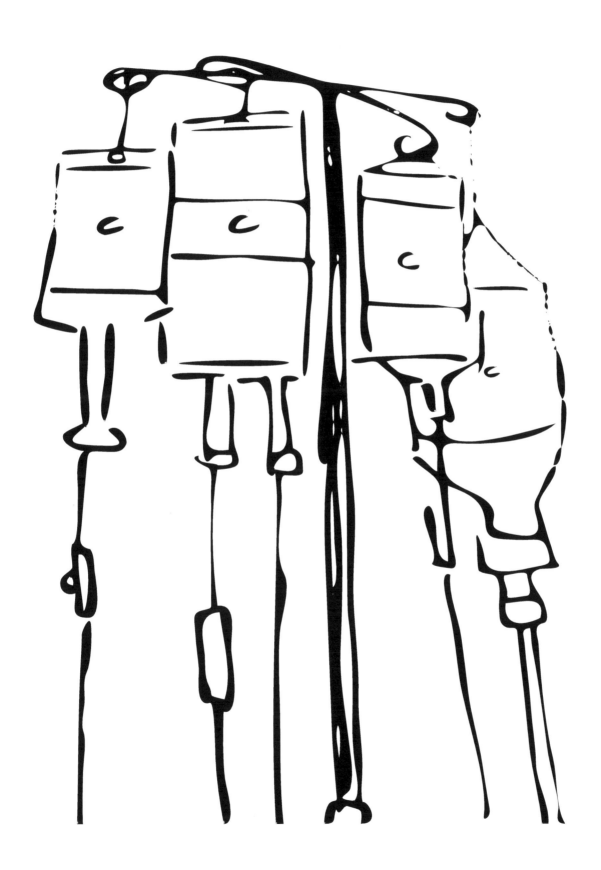

CREATE A LOGO
FOR YOURSELF

HOW ARE "WE" DOING TODAY?

ASSESS THE HIGHLIGHTS OF YOUR DAY.
USE THE SCALE OF 1 TO F.U.!

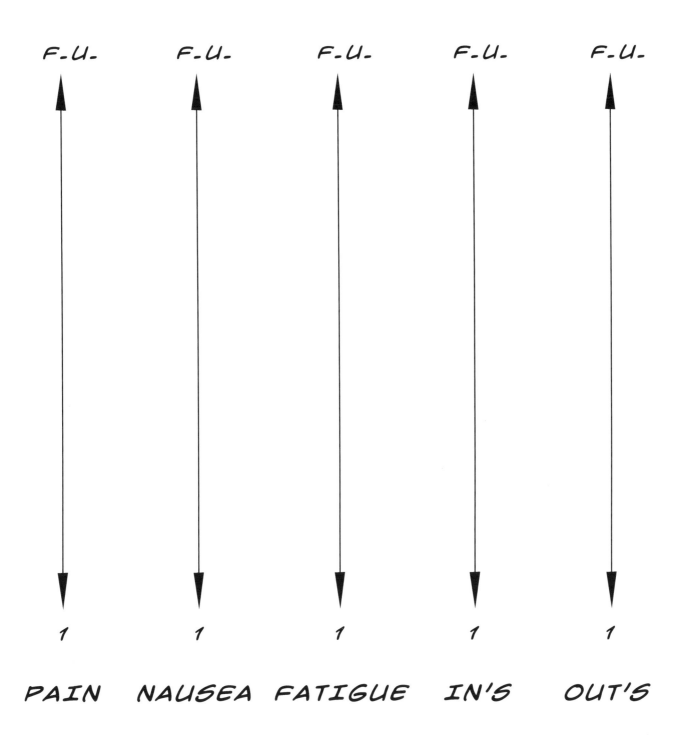

WHAT WOULD YOU DO IF YOU WON THE LOTTERY?

PRACTICE MAKES PERFECT

CANCER PICKED THE WRONG PERSON.

HELLO MY NAME IS CANCER.

HELLO MY NAME IS

HELLO MY NAME IS

HELLO MY NAME IS

HELLO MY NAME IS

HELLO MY NAME IS

HELLO MY NAME IS

HELLO MY NAME IS

HELLO MY NAME IS

DRAW YOUR FAMILY TREE

AMAZE YOURSELF

SCIENCE IS COUNTING ON YOU...

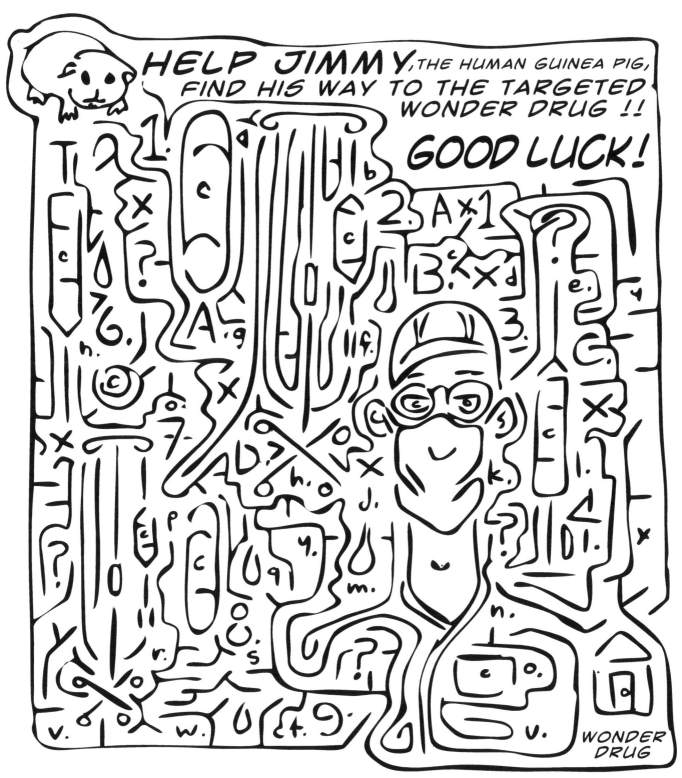

SKETCH YOUR DREAM HOUSE

DOT TO DOT

THIS WON'T HURT A BIT....

1 •• 16

2 •• 15

3 •   •14

C

4 •   5 •• 12   •13

7 •   6 •• 11   •10

8 •   •9

SKETCH YOUR DREAM CAR

CANCER BARBIE

ADD WHAT YOU LIKE !
HAIR STYLE, EYEBROWS, EYE LASHES,
PIERCINGS, CONSTIPATION, HOT FLASHES,
EARRINGS, NAUSEA, FACIAL HAIR, SUNGLASSES...

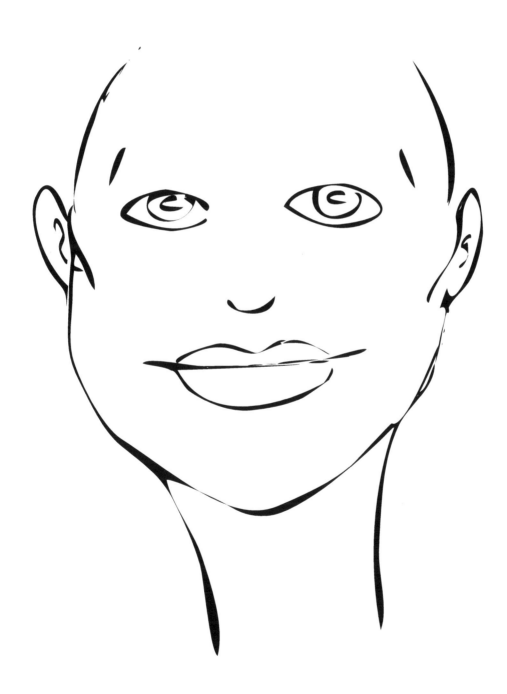

27

LIST NAMES
YOU'D USE AS AN ALIAS

CANCER KEN

ADD WHAT YOU LIKE !
HAIR STYLE, EYEBROWS, NOSE HAIRS, EAR HAIRS
FACIAL HAIR, ERECTILE DYSFUNCTION,
FATIGUE, EYE GLASSES, TATTOOS, WARTS, SCALES...

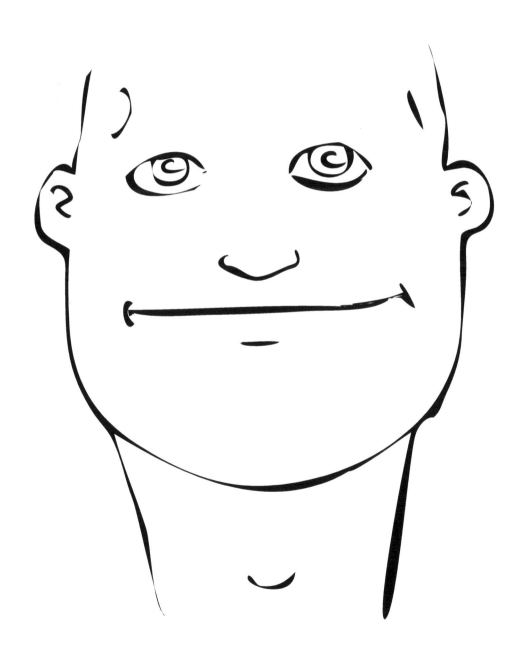

WRITE A SONG
ABOUT CANCER

CANCER FUN

MAKE AS MANY WORDS & PHRASES
AS YOU POSSIBLY CAN. THE FIRST PHRASE IS EASY.

USE THE ADDITIONAL LETTERS FOR EXTRA CREDIT

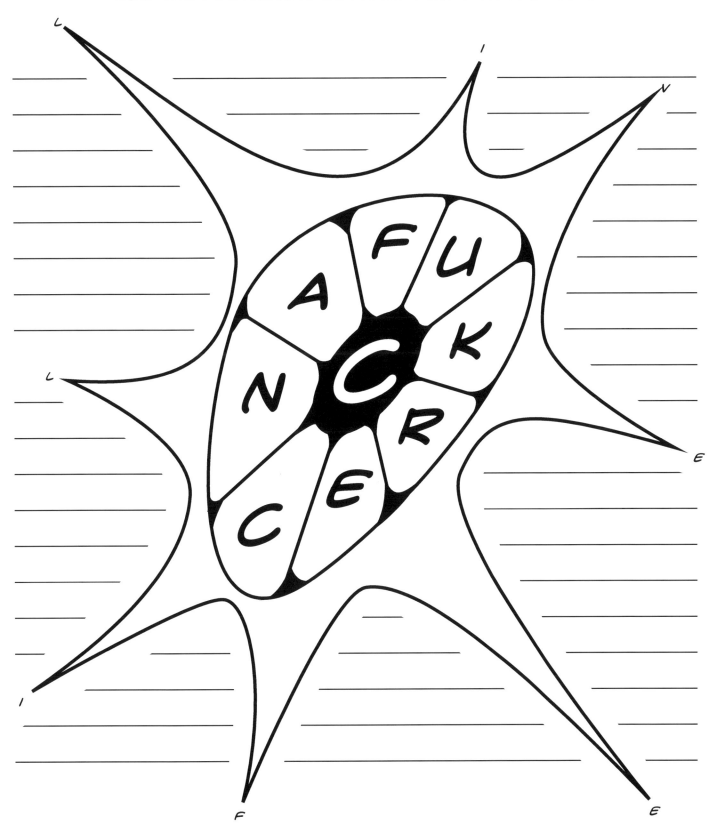

LIST YOUR FAVORITE FUNNY MOVIES

TAKE YOUR TIME TO FIND ALL THE WORDS.
LEFT, RIGHT, UP AND DOWN,
FORWARD AND BACKWARD, TOO.

SKETCH YOURSELF BEFORE AND AFTER CANCER

DOT TO DOT

IT'S GETTING HOT IN HERE!

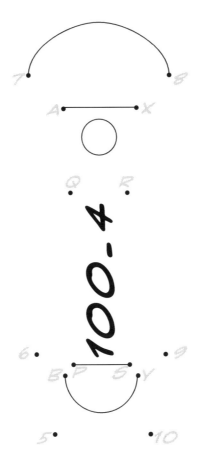

LIST THE INGREDIENTS
IN YOUR CHEMO COCKTAIL

WHOSE I.V. IS IT?

OH BOY, THINGS HAVE BECOME PRETTY TWISTED...
NO NURSES ARE AROUND TO HELP,
IT'S UP TO YOU TO UNTANGLE THIS MESS!

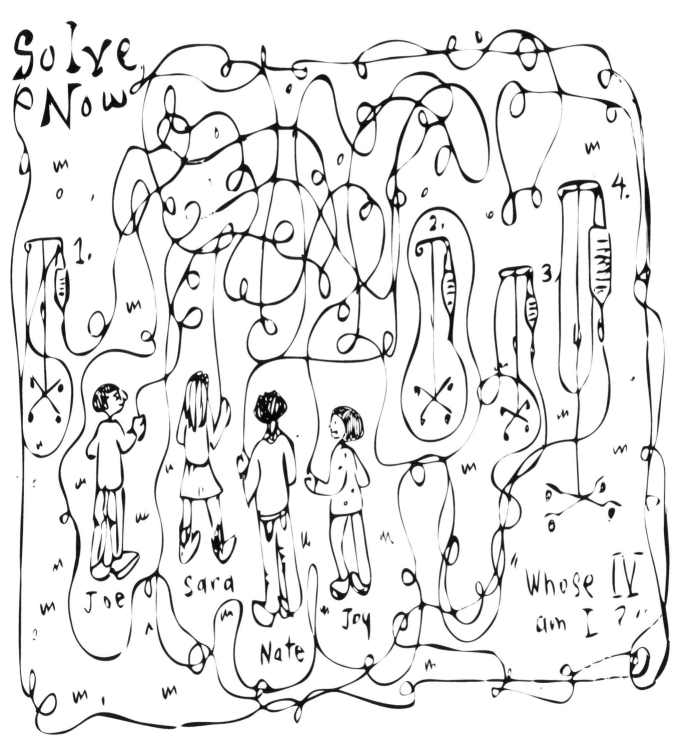

CREATE AN ALBUM COVER
FOR YOUR NEW BAND

HOSPITAL HANGMAN

HINT: NO BARTENDER NEEDED FOR
THIS TYPE OF INFUSION.

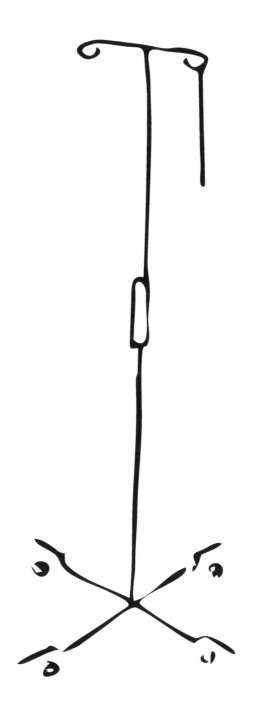

_ _ _ _ T _ _ _ _ _ _ _ _

LIST YOUR FAVORITE FUNNY BOOKS

ALMOST TWINS

SHERRY AND SHARIE ARE SUCH GOOD
FRIENDS AND HANG OUT SO MUCH, THEY
ARE OFTEN MISTAKEN FOR TWINS.
CAN YOU IDENTIFY THEIR DIFFERENCES ?

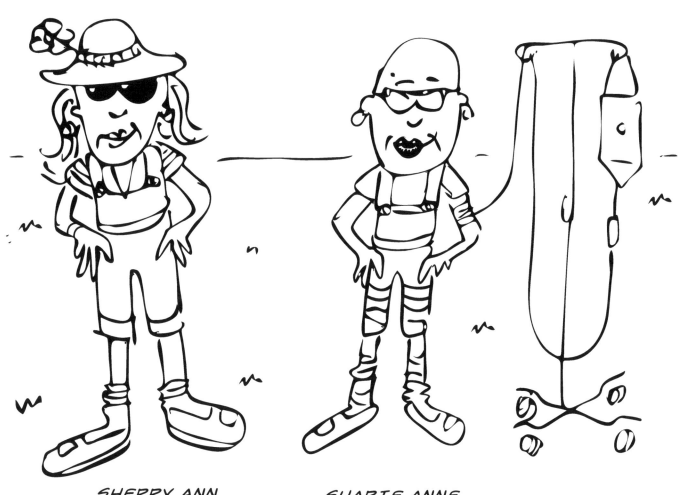

SHERRY ANN
STEPHENS

SHARIE ANNE
STEVENS

FIND THEM ALL

1 _____
2 _____
3 _____
4 _____
5 _____
6 _____

7 _____
8 _____
9 _____
10 _____
11 _____
12 _____

LIST YOUR FAVORITE
SIDE EFFECTS

PRACTICE MAKES PERFECT

MAKE A WISH!

I WISH CANCER WOULD GET CANCER.

I WISH CANCER WOULD

I WISH CANCER WOULD

I WISH CANCER WOULD

I WISH CANCER WOULD

I WISH CANCER WOULD

I WISH CANCER WOULD

I WISH CANCER WOULD

I WISH CANCER WOULD

LIST THE FOODS
THAT TASTE HORRIBLE NOW

LOOK ON THE BRIGHT SIDE

BECAUSE OF CANCER, YOU'LL MASTER A NEW LANGUAGE!
SOLVE EACH ONE, THEN ASSEMBLE THE CIRCLED
LETTERS TO SOLVE THE PHRASE.

_ _ _ _ _ _ _

_ _ (_) _ _ _ _ _ (_)
    2   3

_ (_) _
  4

_ _ _ _ _ _ _ _ _

_ (_) _ _ _ _ _ _
 5

_ _ _ _ _ (_) _
         6

_ _ (_)(_) _
   7 8

(_) _ _ _ _ _ _ _ (_) _ _ _
9   10

_ _ _ _ _ _ (_)
          11

(_) _ _ _
12

_ _ _ _ _

_ _ (_) _ _ _ _ _
   13

NEIAMA

IMOABREKSR

TROP

CONOGSITLO

ATIARDOIN

RGUSERY

UTORM

COMAHERTPYEH

SISEMRNIO

RESMU

OSBIYP

TRVNIANOUES

H _ _ _ _ _   F _ _   _ _ _ C _ _ !
  2   3   4   5   6   7   8   9 10 11   12 13

45

CREATE A NEW
SIGNATURE FOR YOURSELF

HELP THE NEW NURSE

GRAB YOUR CRAYONS AND COLOR IN THE CORRECT MEDS FOR YOUR TREATMENT.

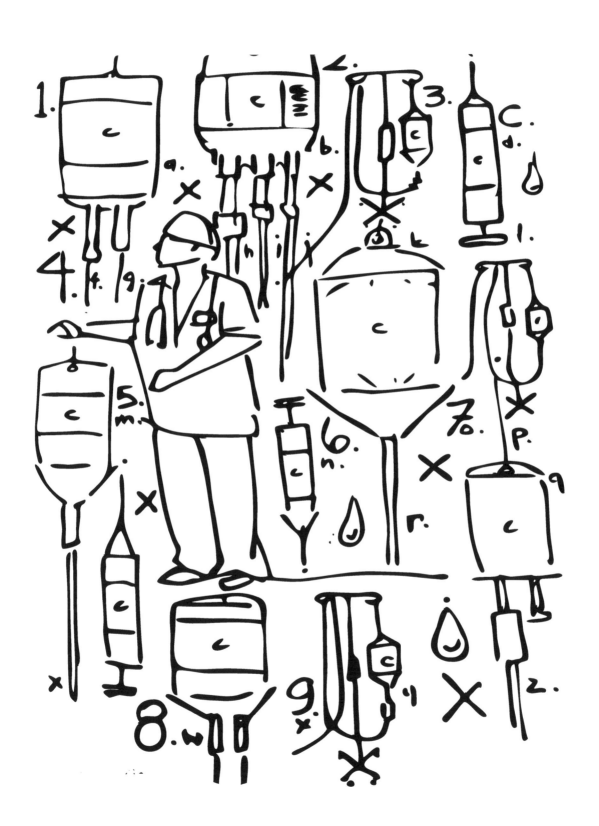

CAMMO CHEMO COLOR CHALLENGE FOR EXTRA CREDIT

DRAW YOUR ALTER-EGO

MR. HYDE COLOR CHALLENGE FOR EXTRA CREDIT

THE HALLS ARE ALIVE !!

WITH THE SOUND OF MUSIC, LOVE AND JOY.

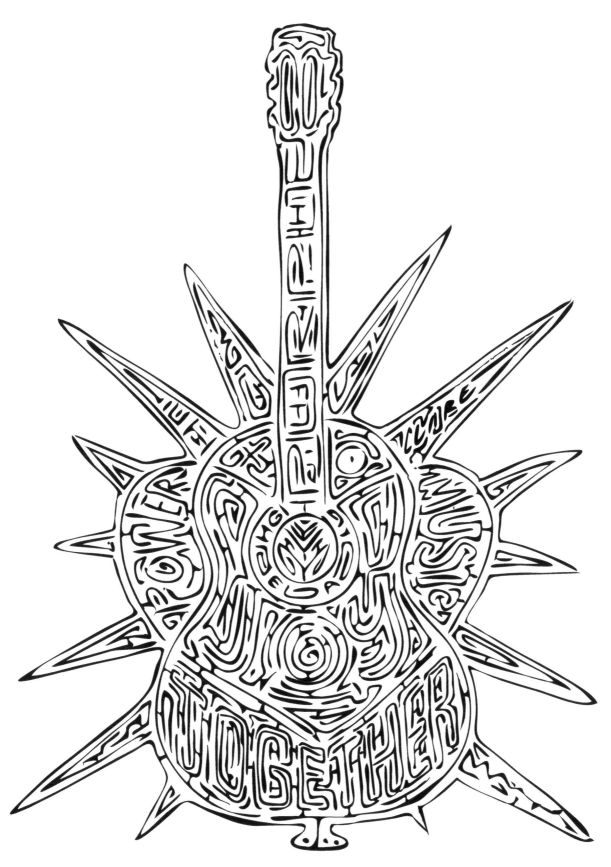

PURPLEZ COLOR CHALLENGE FOR EXTRA CREDIT

WRITE A LETTER
TO YOURSELF

AMAZE YOURSELF

REV UP YOUR RADIOACTIVE EYESIGHT AND FIND YOUR WAY TO THE OTHER SIDE.

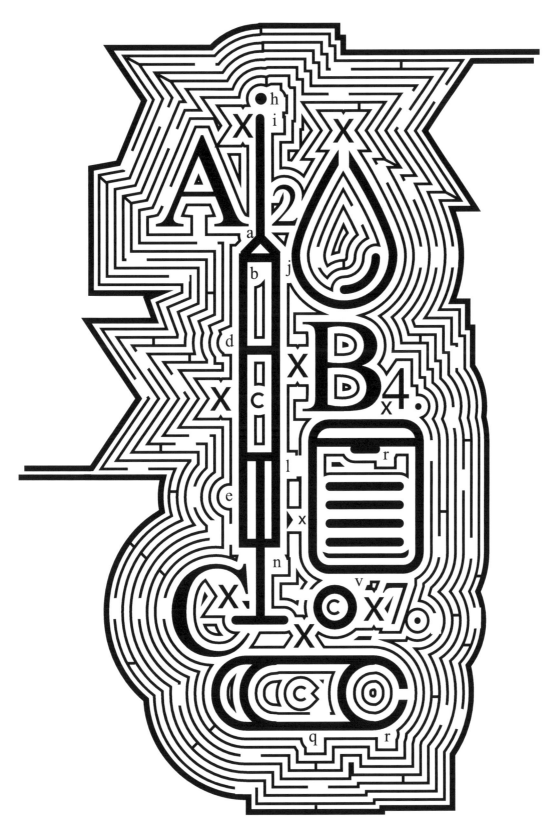

LIST YOUR FAVORITE MEDICAL TERMS

DOT TO DOT

DRIP, DROP, DRIP...

9··10

8·
·A   X·   ·11

C

·B   Y·
7·   ·12

6· ·13

5 14
4···· ··15

3·· ··16
2 17

1· ·18

LIST YOUR
TOP-SECRET SECRETS

LET'S DOSE

ARE YOU LUCID ENOUGH TO ORGANIZE YOUR PILLS THE SAME EACH WEEK?

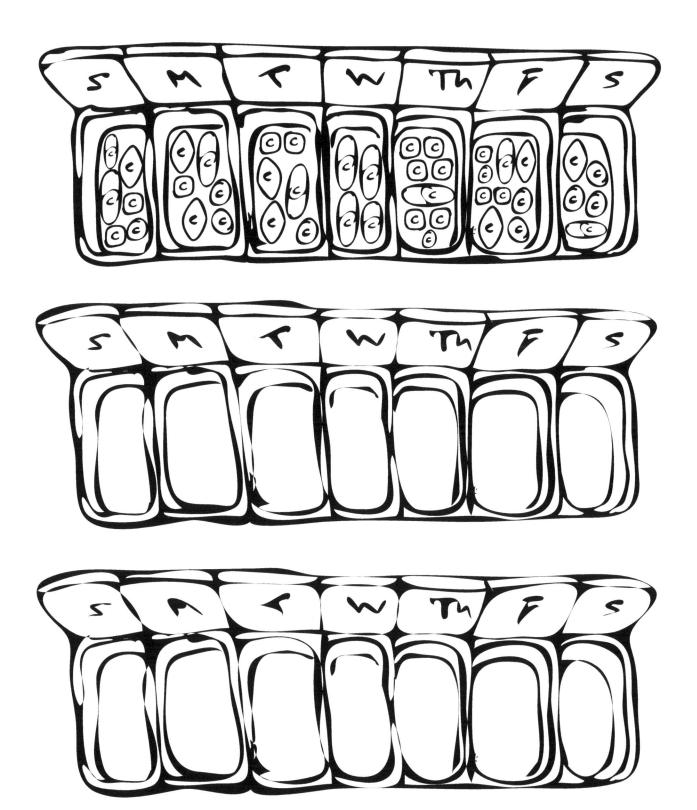

CANDY COLOR CHALLENGE FOR EXTRA CREDIT

SKETCH YOUR
DREAM DATE

PRECISION MEDICINE

FILL IN THE BLANKS

(TO BE READ WITH VIM AND VIGOR)

EVERY _____ DISEASE IS DIFFERENT.
                    EXPLETIVE

INDIVIDUAL _____ APPOINTMENTS HELP OUR _____
                    SAME EXPLETIVE   SAME EXPLETIVE

DOCTORS UNDERSTAND A PATIENT'S _____ DISEASE
                                    SAME EXPLETIVE

AT THE MOLECULAR LEVEL. INFORMATION ABOUT _____
                                                SAME EXPLETIVE

CHANGES THAT ARE UNIQUE TO YOUR _____ DISEASE
                                    SAME EXPLETIVE

WILL HELP US DETERMINE _____ TREATMENTS MOST
                            SAME EXPLETIVE

LIKELY TO WORK FOR _____ EVER !
                        SAME EXPLETIVE

IT IS THE PROMISE OF PRECISION TREATMENT — A FOCUS ON THE

INDIVIDUAL _____ PATIENT.
                SAME EXPLETIVE

WHAT MEDICATIONS WOULD YOU INVENT?

DOT TO DOT

YOUR FEARLESS LEADER...

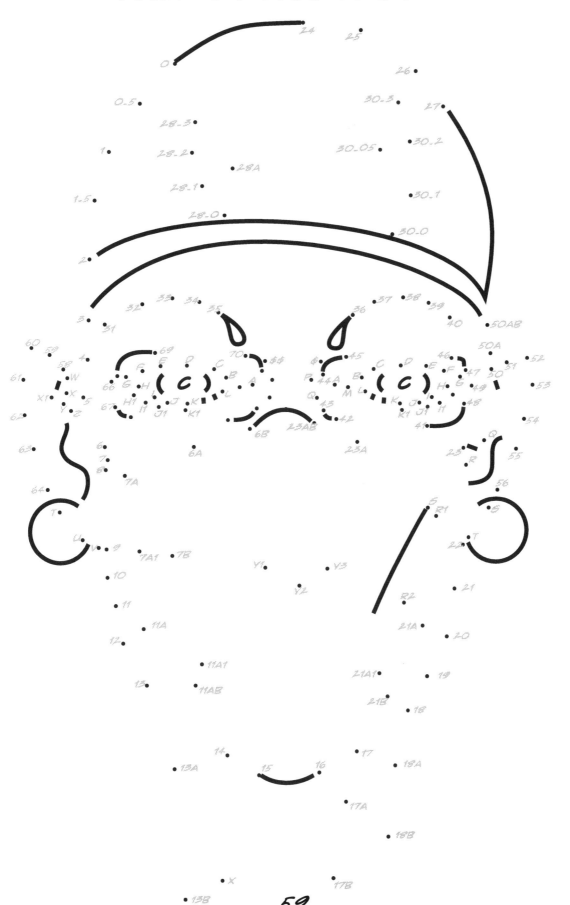

WRITE A LETTER TO AN EVIL VILLIAN

MAZE TIME

GO FROM BEGINNING TO END
BY DRAWING A PATH THROUGH THIS MAZE.
WATCH OUT FOR TRICKY TWISTS AND TURNS.
EVEN TRICKIER THAN SIDE EFFECTS!

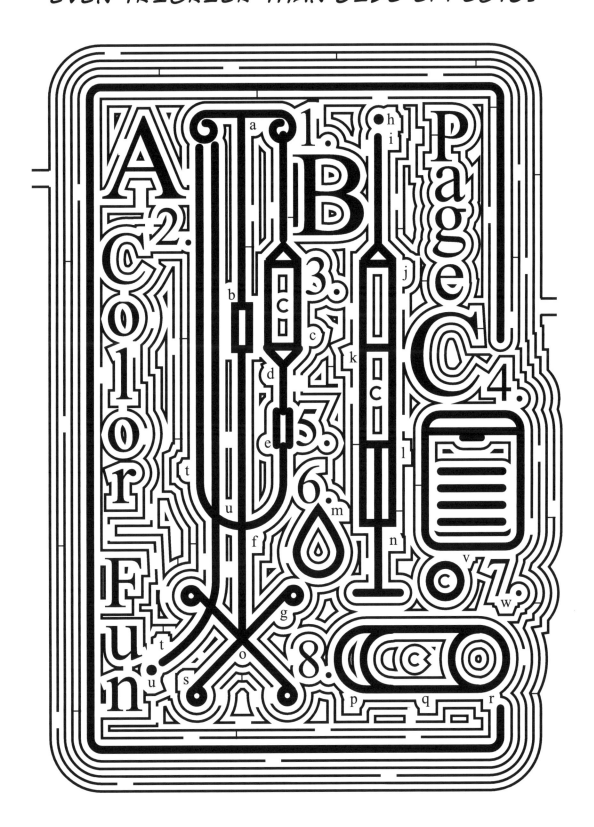

WRITE A LETTER TO YOUR FRIENDS/FAMILY

TOP TEN

REASONS NOT TO BREAK UP WITH SOMEONE WHO HAS CANCER!
RATE THEM 1 – 10

◯

'CHEMO CHIC' IS SO IN

◯

REALLY INTO 'UNTIL DEATH DO US PART'

◯

HOSPITAL BEDS ARE SO INTIMATE

◯

HATES 'LAST TANGO IN PARIS' BUSH

◯

FREE ROOM SERVICE

◯

LIKES A CHALLENGE

◯

HATES CASUAL RELATIONSHIPS

◯

LOVES PLAYING 'DOCTOR'

◯

LATEX FETISH

◯

CANCER IS SEXY

WRITE A HAIKU
ABOUT CANCER

TREATMENT WORD FIND

FIND THEM ALL
FORWARD AND BACKWARD, UP AND DOWN.
THEN COMBINE DARKENED LETTERS
TO GET YOUR PROGNOSIS.

```
c  l  v  x  i  v  x  A  c  i  n  i  L  c  o  h
h  a  n  e  m  i  a  P  o  w  e  r  m  x  h  o
e  o  e     m  R  e  m  i  s  s  i  o  n  e  p
m  x  u  c  u  c  l  x  w  H  i  v  n  r  m  E
o  y  t  y  n  a  i  e  o  e  i  x  o  r  o  y
t  g  r  c  e  n  g  v  r  a  o  m  c  i  g  o
h  r  o  i  s  c  h  o  r  i  v  e  y  c  l  u
e  e  p  e  y  r  t  l  a  e  e  x  t  k  o  v
r  n  h  s  s  e  r  u  m  r  k  o  e  x  b  l
a  e  l  v  t  r  P  l  a  t  e  l  e  t  i  v
p  o  l  m  e  s  i  c  k  n  e  s  s  x  h  l
y  T  X  e  m  s  r  e  k  r  a  m  o  l  b  v
y  R  A  D  i  a  T  i  o  N  x  m  e  v  r  d
i  o  x  i  v  o  o  v  D  o  c  T  o  R  v
v  P  l  o  v  e  x  s  u  r  g  e  v  y  k  y
H  o  s  p  i  T  s  i  l  e  c  e  T  i  w
```

H _ _ _ _ _   _ _ _ _ _ _

LIST EVERYONE YOU'VE EVER SLEPT WITH

GRAMPIE CAN'T FLY !

TREATMENT ONLY GROUNDED GRAMPIE'S BODY...
BUT HIS IMAGINATION STILL LETS HIM FLY!!!

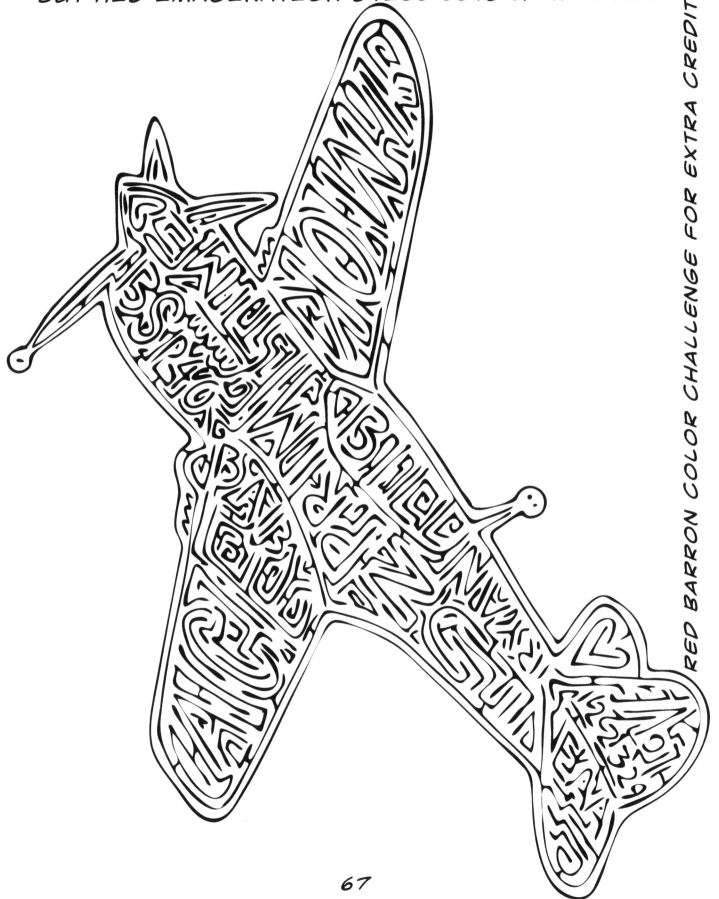

RED BARRON COLOR CHALLENGE FOR EXTRA CREDIT

LIST THE PLACES
YOU WANT TO CONQUER

DOCTORS NIGHT OFF

THIS DOCTOR HAS HAD A BUSY WEEK HELPING
KICK CANCERS ASS. NOW IT'S YOUR TURN TO HELP
HIM DRESS UP FOR A NIGHT OUT ON THE TOWN!

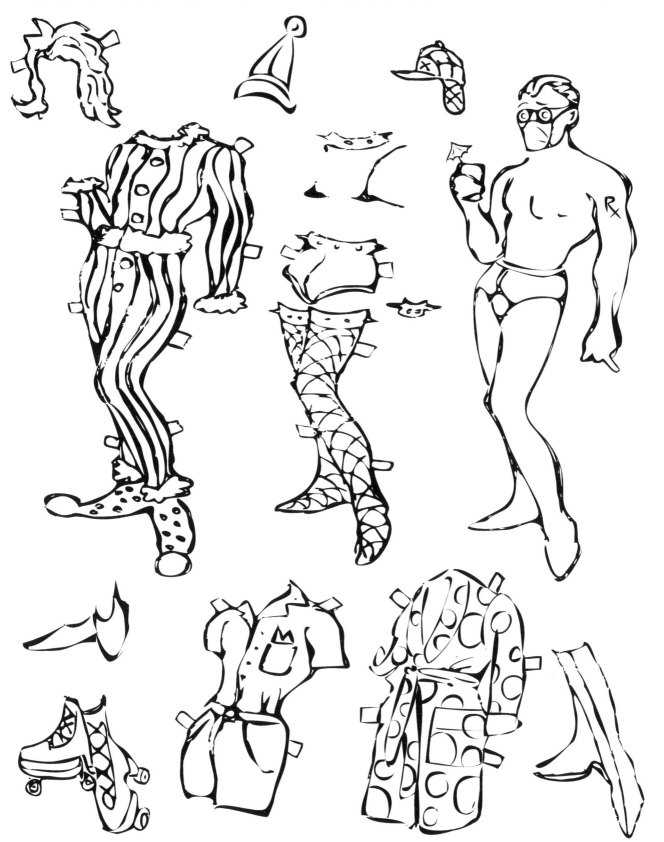

SWANKY COLOR CHALLENGE FOR EXTRA CREDIT

WRITE A LETTER TO YOUR INSURANCE COMPANY

THE GRASS IS GREEN

COLOR AND DRIVE YOUR CARES AWAY.....
FORE!!

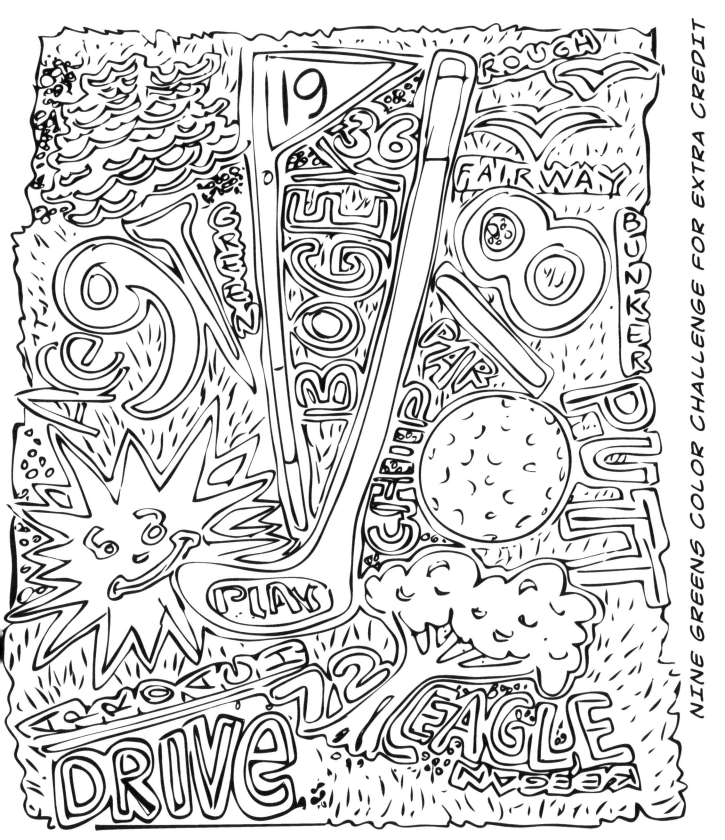

HOW MANY NURSES CAN YOU GET TO SIGN THIS PAGE?

TOP TEN

A MULLIGAN IS A GOLF TERM FOR A DO-OVER.
WHAT WOULD YOUR CANCER MULLIGANS BE?

RATE THEM 1 — 10

○ CHEMO MULLIGAN

○ MED MULLIGAN

○ SURGICAL MULLIGAN

○ BED PAN MULLIGAN

○ RADIATION MULLIGAN

○ DIAGNOSIS MULLIGAN

○ DR MULLIGAN

○ TUMOR MULLIGAN

○ ANY HOLE MULLIGAN

○ TREATMENT MULLIGAN

LIST YOUR
FAVORITE QUOTES

AMAZE YOURSELF

HELP YOUR DOCTOR GET THROUGH THE MAZE OF DATA
TO MAKE THE CORRECT DIAGNOSIS.

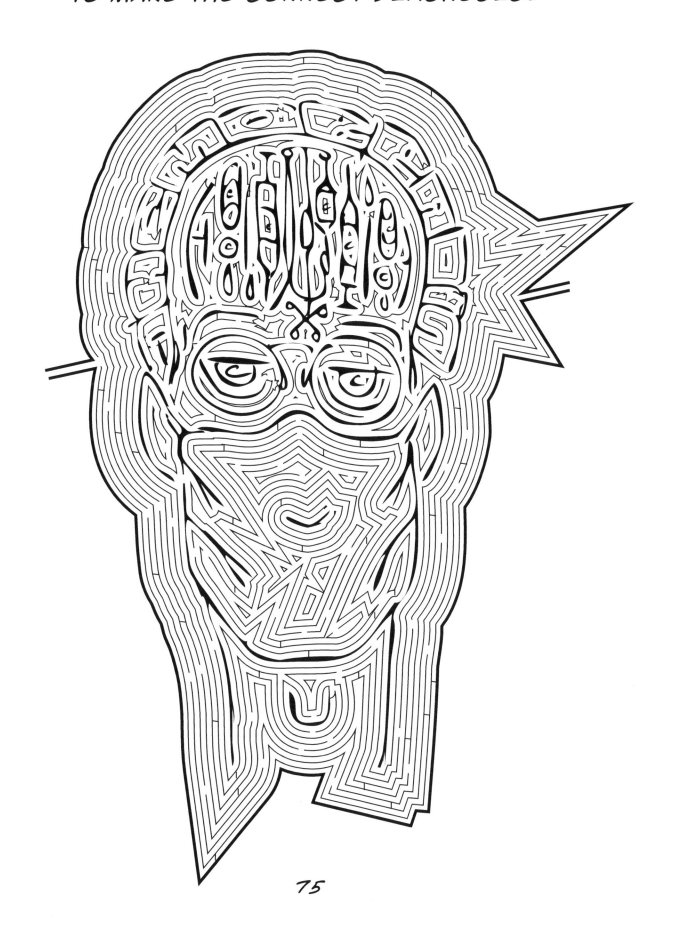

WHAT'S YOUR MOST EMBARASSING MOMENT.... SO FAR?

VISITORS

CREATE LASTING MEMORIES!

NAME	DATE	REMARKS

MUCHLOVE !

Made in the USA
Columbia, SC
27 July 2022